THE LATEST ON MONKEYPOX

With focus on the United States of America

Dr. Jennifer L. Spencer

TABLE OF CONTENTS

Introduction

The monkeypox virus is the cause of the viral zoonotic illness monkeypox. Fever, a severe headache, swollen lymph nodes, throbbing pain in the muscles, and a rash that blisters and crusts are some of the symptoms. The cheeks, palms of the hands, and bottoms of the feet are typically where the rash is concentrated. It may also affect the eyes, lips, and genitalia.

The virus that causes smallpox, the variola virus, is related to the virus that causes monkeypox. The symptoms of monkeypox are comparable to those of smallpox but less severe, and monkeypox rarely results in death. Chickenpox and monkeypox are unrelated.

A person can be contagious throughout the symptoms, which can range from mild to severe and typically linger for many weeks.

Without treatment, the majority of patients recover after a few weeks.

The first case of human monkeypox in humans was discovered in 1970 in the Democratic Republic of the Congo in a 9-month-old boy in an area where smallpox had been eradicated in 1968. Since that time, the majority of human cases have been found in remote, rainforest regions of the Congo Basin, mainly in the Democratic Republic of the Congo, and cases have spread across central and west Africa.

In addition to affecting nations in west and central Africa, monkeypox has a significant impact on worldwide public health. The first monkeypox outbreak outside of Africa occurred in the United States in 2003 and was attributed to contact with pet prairie dogs who were infected.

These animals had been housed alongside imported dormice and pouched rats from Ghana that were from the Gambia. In the U.S., this outbreak caused more than 70 cases of monkeypox. Explorers from Nigeria have likewise announced instances of monkeypox in Israel in September 2018, the United Kingdom in September 2018, December 2019, May 2021, and May 2022, Singapore in May 2019, and the United States between July and November, 2021. Monkeypox outbreaks were reported in many non-endemic nations in May 2022. To further understand the epidemiology, sources of infection, and patterns of transmission, studies are now being conducted.

The pathogen

The Orthopoxvirus genus of the Poxviridae family includes the double-stranded DNA virus known as the monkeypox virus, which is enclosed.

The monkeypox virus has two distinct genetic clades, one in central Africa (Congo Basin), and the other in west Africa. In the past, the Congo Basin clade was thought to be more contagious and to produce more severe illnesses. Cameroon, which forms the physical divide between the two groups, is the only country where both viral clades have been identified.

Transmission

Direct contact with the blood, body fluids and cutaneous or mucosal lesions of infected animals can result in animal-to-human (zoonotic) transfer. Infection with the monkeypox virus has been detected in a large number of African animals, including rope squirrels, tree squirrels, Gambian pouched rats, dormice, and numerous kinds of monkeys.

Although it has not yet been determined, rodents are the most likely candidates for the monkeypox natural reservoir. Consuming raw meat and other infected animal products can increase risk. Living near or in forests can expose people to ill animals inadvertently or minimally.

Human-to-human transmission may be triggered by close contact with respiratory secretions, skin lesions on an infected person, or recently contaminated objects. Because droplet respiratory particles often necessitate prolonged face-to-face contact, health professionals, families, and other close contacts of current patients are more at risk. The longest reported chain of transmission within a community has shown an increase from 6 to 9 person-to-person infections.

This may signal a general loss in immunity brought on by the cessation of smallpox vaccination programs. Transmission through the placenta, which can also occur during close contact during labor and after birth, can result in congenital monkeypox. Although intimate physical contact is a known risk factor for transmission, it is still unknown if sexual activity specifically contributes to the spread of monkeypox. Studies are necessary to fully understand this risk.

Signs and symptoms

Monkeypox typically takes 6 to 13 days to incubate, although it can take anything from 5 to 21 days for symptoms to appear.

The infection goes through two stages:

1. Fever, severe headache, lymphadenopathy (swelling of the lymph nodes), back discomfort, myalgia (muscle aches), and severe asthenia are all symptoms of the 0–5-

day invasion period (lack of energy). When compared to other illnesses that could at first appear similar, monkeypox has a distinctive feature called lymphadenopathy (chickenpox, measles, smallpox)

2. Typically, the skin eruption starts 1-3 days after the onset of fever. The rash typically appears on the face and limbs rather than the trunk. The face is affected in 95% of instances, while the palms of the hands and the bottoms of the feet are affected in 75% of cases. In 70% of cases, the conjunctiva, oral mucous membranes, and genitalia are also affected in addition to the cornea. From macules, which are flat, firm lesions, the rash progresses to papules, which are slightly raised, firm lesions, vesicles, which are clear fluid-filled lesions, pustules, which are yellowish fluid-filled lesions, and crusts that dry up and break off. The number of lesions

can be somewhere between a few and several thousand. In severe cases, lesions may merge, resulting in large portions of skin flaking off.

Monkeypox often has symptoms that last between two and four weeks and is a self-limiting condition. Due to the level of viral exposure, the patient's health, and the nature of the issues, children are more prone to encounter severe cases. In the event of immunological impairments, the outcomes might be severe. Although smallpox vaccination provided protection in the past, the worldwide cessation of smallpox vaccination campaigns after the disease was eradicated may have made people under the age of 40 to 50 (depending on the country) more vulnerable to monkeypox. Secondary infections, bronchopneumonia, sepsis, encephalitis, and corneal infections with resultant vision loss are some of the problems associated with monkeypox.

How widespread an asymptomatic infection might be is unknown.

The case fatality ratio of monkeypox has historically ranged from 0 to 11% in the general population; it has been greater among small children. Recently, the case mortality rate was between 3 and 6 percent.

Diagnosis

When making a clinical differential diagnosis, it is important to include other rash disorders such chickenpox, measles, bacterial skin infections, scabies, syphilis, and allergies caused by prescription medications. Lymphadenopathy at the prodromal stage of the illness can help distinguish monkeypox from chickenpox or smallpox as a clinical feature.

Health professionals should get the right sample and arrange for it to be delivered safely to a lab with the right equipment if monkeypox is detected.

The kind of laboratory test used and the type and quality of the specimen used determine whether monkeypox is confirmed.

As a result, specimens should be sent and handled in line with local, state, and federal regulations. Given its precision and sensitivity, polymerase chain reaction (PCR) is the primary laboratory test. The best diagnostic samples for monkeypox come from skin lesions, such as dry crusts and the liquid that comes from vesicles and pustules. The biopsy is a possibility when it is possible. Lesion samples must be maintained cool and stored in a dry, sterile tube without a viral transport medium. Due to the short period of viremia about the date of specimen collection after symptoms begin, PCR blood tests are typically inconclusive and should not be regularly obtained from patients.

Antigen and antibody detection techniques do not offer proof of monkeypox-specific infection because orthopoxviruses are serologically cross-reactive. Therefore, in cases where resources are scarce, serology and antigen detection procedures are not advised for diagnosis or case inquiry. Furthermore, recent or distant immunization with a vaccinia-based vaccine (for example, anyone immunized before the eradication of smallpox, or more recently due to heightened risk, such as orthopoxvirus laboratory employees) may result in false positive results.

The following patient data must be included with the specimens to interpret test results:

a) age;

b) date of onset of fever;

c) date of the specimen collection;

d) date of the current condition of the patient (stage of rash), and

e) date of the beginning of the rash.

<u>Therapeutics</u>

To treat monkeypox symptoms effectively, handle complications, and avoid long-term effects, clinical care must be properly optimized. Fluids and food should be provided to patients to maintain a healthy nutritional condition. Bacterial secondary infections should be treated as necessary. The European Medicines Agency (EMA) authorized the use of tecovirimat, a smallpox treatment medicine, to treat monkeypox in 2022 on the basis of data from both animal and human research. It still isn't easily reachable.

If tecovirimat is utilized for patient treatment, it is ideal to monitor it in a clinical research setting with prospective data gathering.

How smallpox and monkeypox are related

Monkeypox shares several clinical characteristics with smallpox, a closely related but now-extinct orthopoxvirus illness. Smallpox was more frequently lethal and easier to spread because roughly 30% of patients died from it. After a worldwide vaccination and containment campaign, the last naturally occurring case of smallpox occurred in 1977, and smallpox was deemed to be eradicated worldwide in 1980. Since all nations stopped administering vaccinia-based vaccinations for routine smallpox vaccination, it has been at least 40 years. Unvaccinated populations are now more vulnerable to infection with the monkeypox virus because vaccination also protected monkeypox in west and central Africa.

Although smallpox is no longer naturally occurring, the global health industry is nonetheless on high alert in case it should resurface due to natural mechanisms, laboratory accidents, or malicious intent.

To ensure that the entire world is prepared in the event that smallpox returns, newer vaccines, diagnostics, and antiviral medications are being developed. Now, these might be used to treat and prevent monkeypox.

The monkeypox virus's natural host

The monkeypox virus is susceptible to several animal species. In addition to non-human primates, dormice, rope and tree squirrels, Gambian pouched rats, and other species are included. The natural history of the monkeypox virus is still unknown, and more investigation is needed to identify the precise reservoir or reservoirs and comprehend how the virus spreads in the wild.

U.S. cases of monkeypox

On May 18, 2022, the first case of the current monkeypox outbreak in the United States was discovered. As of July 26, 3,591 cases had been located in 46 states, Puerto Rico, and Washington, D.C.; this represents 19% of the 19,188 cases that had been formally confirmed globally. The stigma that may prevent people from seeking medical care, especially when sores are in the genital or anal region and transmission may be linked to same-sex sexual encounters, are some of the reasons why this number is likely significantly undercounted. Other reasons include limited access to testing, especially in the early months of the outbreak; a delay between seeing a provider and having a case confirmed; knowledge gaps among providers; and stigma.

On July 23, 2022, the World Health Organization (WHO) announced that the monkeypox outbreak was a Public Health Emergency of International

Concern (PHEIC) because of the growing number of cases and other factors.

The WHO also offered a list of suggestions for what governments and other parties can do to combat the outbreak. It remains to be seen whether the United States will follow suit and declare the epidemic to be a domestic PHE. If money were required, doing so would provide several flexibilities. In the upcoming weeks, confirmed cases are anticipated to increase further, most likely as a result of both an actual spike in cases brought on by continued transmission and advancements in testing.

Gay, bisexual, and other men who have sex with men are currently thought to be the most at risk and have accounted for nearly all recorded cases in the current U.S. outbreak. In the current outbreak, cases have been found among transgender men and cisgender women.

However, monkeypox can be a risk for anyone, regardless of sexual orientation or the sex or gender of sexual partners.

The virus has two strains: a less harmful west African variant that is causing the present outbreak in the United States, and a more severe central African (Congo Basin) strain. Although the infection can be severe, the majority of cases in the U.S. have been minor to date, and the majority of hospitalizations have been used to manage discomfort. However, reports of myocarditis and encephalopathy linked to monkeypox have also been made.

Its incubation period lasts for one to two weeks, and the symptoms that manifest first after the incubation period may be those that are typical of a variety of viral infections, such as:

bodily aches, fatigue, a fever, a headache, and enlarged lymph nodes.

Lesions and a severe rash are frequently next. Even though lesions can develop anywhere on the body (for example, on the hands, feet, chest, or eyes), in the most recent epidemic, they have frequently been discovered in the anal and vaginal regions, which can be uncomfortable. Serious illnesses are more likely to affect those with compromised immune systems, which may include HIV-positive individuals who are not virally suppressed.

The illness usually lasts between two and four weeks.

Direct contact with lesions, rashes, scabs, or fluids that are infected can spread monkeypox between individuals. Although some virus has been found in samples, it is unknown if semen or vaginal fluid can also transmit the disease;

exposure to contaminated objects, such as clothing or linens;

respiratory aerosols from extended face-to-face contact (unlike COVID-19, monkeypox is not believed to be transmitted via respiratory aerosols); and placenta-to-fetus transmission in pregnant women.

Once symptoms appear, those who have monkeypox are contagious to others and stay contagious until lesions develop scabs, scabs break off, and a new layer of skin grows. Monkeypox patients are advised to remain isolated until this time, which may take up to 4 weeks. Monkeypox sufferers can take preventative measures to reduce their risk of spreading the disease to others, such as avoiding close contact with others, including sexual activity, and refraining from sharing possibly contaminated things including dishware, clothes, linens, and towels.

When did the U.S. federal government start responding to the outbreak?

The CDC and other agencies took initial response measures after the first cases of this outbreak of monkeypox were discovered (in the United Kingdom on May 6, 2022, and in the United States on May 18, 2022). These actions included creating an updated case definition for monkeypox, giving guidance to local, state, tribal, and territorial health departments on surveillance, reporting, and contact tracing, supporting diagnostic testing, and coordinating with international authorities and other countries.

The CDC activated its Emergency Operations Center to improve operational support, including monitoring and coordination, and the White House announced a government-wide strategy and approach to scaling up vaccination and expanding testing capacity for monkeypox on June 28, 2022, six weeks after the first case of the disease in the United States.

The administration's reaction has drawn criticism from certain public health professionals and campaigners who claim that the government did not move quickly or broadly enough and is now playing "catch up" in crucial response areas including messaging and extending access to immunizations, tests, and treatments. Some people voiced concern that the federal government is making the same mistakes it did in its first response to the COVID-19 pandemic and warned that the monkeypox outbreak might swiftly grow even larger if more testing, vaccinations, and particular precautions are not taken. According to the administration, when the situation changes, the nation's response will also be modified.

What areas are the U.S. response's primary focus?

Responding to epidemics as the monkeypox epidemic falls under the purview of both the federal government and the state, municipal, and tribal governments.

The federal government's response has thus far concentrated on several areas, including:

1. vaccines and treatments
2. conducting and improving surveillance
3. expanding testing accessibility and capacity
4. educating healthcare professionals and the public
5. supporting research and development; coordinating with and supporting state, local, and territorial responses
6. developing and pursuing research priorities; and engaging with affected communities and other stakeholders.

Many of these initiatives are also supported by state and local governments, with help from the federal government. For instance, some jurisdictions are striving to make it easier for medical professionals to get tested, treated, and immunized, as well as helping to spread important information about the outbreak and build local response networks. However, these responses vary across the nation and are stronger in certain regions than others.

Which federal agencies are a part of the response?

The U.S. Department of Health and Human Services (HHS) and a number of its operating divisions and offices are involved in the federal response, which is coordinated by the White House National Security Council's Directorate on Global Health Security and Biodefense (also known as the White House Pandemic Preparedness Office).

These include the CDC, the Food and Drug Administration (FDA), the National Institutes of Health, and the Office of the Assistant Secretary for Preparedness and Response (ASPR, which houses the Strategic National Stockpile under the Office of Operations and Resources as well as the Biomedical Advanced Research and Development Authority (BARDA) (NIH). A part is also played by the White House Office of Science and Technology Policy (OSTP).

How far along is the American monkeypox testing program?

Only a select group of authorized laboratories are currently able to conduct monkeypox testing, and testing capacity has gradually increased. Clinical samples taken from patients' lesions are tested for the presence of an Orthopoxvirus or, in some cases, specifically the monkeypox virus.

Initially, public health laboratories like the CDC and others were the main locations for testing. Testing has more recently been extended to private laboratories:

By June 28, 2022, there were 78 labs (mainly public health labs) in 48 states with the ability to test 10,000 orthopoxvirus samples each week, up from 67 labs with a capacity of 8,000 samples per week two years earlier.

To increase testing capacity and improve accessibility for providers and patients, HHS announced on June 22, 2022, that it had started shipping CDC Orthopoxvirus tests to five commercial laboratory companies - Aegis Science, Labcorp, Mayo Clinic Laboratories, Quest Diagnostics, and Sonic Healthcare.

The CDC Orthopoxvirus test was being used by Aegis Science, Labcorp, the Mayo Clinic Laboratories, and Sonic Healthcare as of July 18.

Each of these labs can perform up to 10,000 tests per week.

Since then, Quest Diagnostics has declared that they have created a test that is only for monkeypox as opposed to the Orthopoxvirus test as a whole and anticipates being able to conduct 30,000 of those tests weekly by the end of July. To provide another testing option, Quest has stated that it will continue to work toward validating the general CDC Orthopoxvirus test. They anticipate that this additional capacity will be available in August.

The capacity of the American public health laboratories and the private sector to test for the orthopoxvirus, or monkeypox virus, is presently 80,000 tests per week.

There have been occasional complaints of difficulties getting access to monkeypox testing, especially before the private labs and the CDC partnered to provide tests. Even though there are now commercial labs that offer the testing, there are still obstacles because not all providers are prepared or willing to collect the specimens. Additionally, tests conducted by commercial laboratories may have costs, which could be problematic for patients who are underinsured or without insurance. In contrast, tests conducted at public health laboratories are free of charge for patients.

How is the supply of monkeypox vaccines doing in the United States?

Monkeypox vaccines can be administered as a preventative measure before exposure occurs (pre-exposure prophylaxis, or PrEP) or as a response to known or anticipated exposure (post-exposure prophylaxis, or PEP).

Vaccines against monkeypox are offered through the Strategic National Stockpile. Only 65,000 JYNNEOS doses were in the stockpile as of late

June, making the U.S. 's supply of such doses currently quite scarce.

More doses have been ordered and will be delivered in the upcoming months, with 6.9 million doses of JYNNEOS (enough to vaccinate 3.5 million individuals) anticipated to be accessible by mid-2023, including roughly 1.9 million doses in 2022. (enough to vaccinate 950,000 people).

Of these, 5.5 million JYNNEOS doses have just been ordered by the American government and are part of a bulk purchase for vaccines that HHS/BARDA has with vaccine manufacturer Bavarian Nordic under an active ten-year contract. The agreement enables the U.S. government to ask Bavarian Nordic to "fill and finish" the number of vaccines it has purchased, which amounts to more than 15 million doses. It is still unknown if the US government intends to purchase any additional JYNNEOS dosages under this arrangement in addition to the 5.5 million doses that have already been made public.

Although the JYNNEOS vaccine is preferred and advised for most, HHS also stated that the strategic national stockpile holds more than 100 million doses of the ACAM2000 vaccine, a smallpox vaccine thought to be effective for monkeypox as well.

Where and how were vaccination doses dispersed?

According to HHS, JYNNEOS doses started to be shipped on May 21, 2022, and as of July 22, 2022, 333,218 doses (93% of which had been shipped) had been distributed to all 50 states as well as seven jurisdictions/groups (American Samoa, Washington, D.C., Guam, the Northern Mariana Islands, Tribal Entities, Puerto Rico, and the U.S. Virgin Islands).

Several sizable cities also received additional dosages on top of the state-specific amounts.

Up to this point, New York has received the most doses, followed by California and Florida.

A "four-tier distribution system that prioritizes countries with the highest incidence rates of monkeypox" is used to distribute JYNNEOS dosages. The number of people at risk for monkeypox who also have pre-existing illnesses, such as HIV, will determine how many doses of JYNNEOS are distributed within each tier. Priority was given to allocating the vaccines first to jurisdictions with a higher number of cases and severely afflicted populations.

Allocations in the present phase have specifically been based on transmission (current and anticipated monkeypox cases) and the prevalence of high-risk populations (i.e. men who have sex with men with HIV or who are eligible for HIV PrEP). Jurisdictions must submit requests to the CDC and, in most circumstances, use funds from their allotments to obtain vaccines. While vaccine supplies are limited, the CDC has advised that vaccinations be given to people with confirmed and suspected monkeypox exposure (as PEP and PEP++, respectively); however, some communities, including New York City and Washington, DC, have made vaccination more widely available to higher risk groups, such as gay and bisexual men and other men who have sex with men.

Additionally, jurisdictions have the option of requesting the ACAM2000 vaccine. As of July 1, according to HHS, these requests led to the distribution of more than 800 doses of ACAM2000.

How is the therapy for monkeypox doing in the United States?

The monkeypox virus is not the target of any therapy currently in use. However, because the viruses that cause smallpox and monkeypox are identical, monkeypox treatments may also work for smallpox. The antiviral Ticoviromat (TPOXX), which has been given smallpox approval, is currently the course of treatment for monkeypox infection in the United States under an expanded access investigational new drug (EA-IND) program. By the end of June 2022, HHS stated that it had deployed 300 courses from the strategic national stockpile, which had over 1.7 million TPOXX antiviral therapy courses (it is unclear where these doses have been distributed).

The CDC must give its users the go-ahead because TPOXX is only accessible through an EA-IND process for the treatment of monkeypox. There have been numerous accounts of clinicians having to go through drawn-out and onerous processes to get their patients the care they need, which puts patients at a disadvantage and presents difficulties for the providers. The CDC announced changes to this procedure on July 22, 2022, in response to these difficulties. Although the CDC still needs to authorize the use of this medication, the approval procedure has been made a little easier by cutting the number of required forms, patient samples, and images & [offering] patients the opportunity to visit their doctor online.

What federal funding is accessible for local governments to combat monkeypox?

Congress hasn't yet allocated any more money or urgent funds just for the monkeypox response. However, the CDC has acknowledged that a number of its current grants are flexible enough to let local governments spend money for monkeypox as required.

Four financing sources have been used in these so far:

1. PHEP financing enables public health departments to "develop and expand their capacities to successfully respond to a range of public health hazards, including infectious diseases, natural disasters, and biological, chemical, nuclear, and radioactive incidents."

2. Increasing STD PCHD (STD Prevention and Control for Health Departments) Cooperation: STD PCHD grants assist grantees in their efforts to combat STDs, particularly in priority populations such as "adolescents and young adults, men who have sex with men, and pregnant women."

3. Following the Epidemiology and Laboratory Capacity (ELC) Building for the Prevention of Emerging Infections Disease Cooperative Agreement, grantee activities "to detect,

respond to, control, and prevent infectious diseases" are supported by ELC financing.

4. Community Health Workers for COVID Response and Resilient Communities (CCR): The CCR program offers to fund for "opportunities intended to place more trained [community health workers] CHWs in communities that have been hardest hit by COVID-19 and among populations at high risk for COVID-19 exposure, infection, and illness."

What public relations and messaging initiatives are being carried out concerning the outbreak?

Messaging aimed at this community is particularly crucial, especially when it takes into account the stigma and discrimination these communities encounter. This monkeypox outbreak has disproportionately affected gay, bisexual, and other men who have sex with men. To alert them about the developing monkeypox outbreak and to offer recommendations on illness presentation, development, testing, and treatment, HHS has been contacting the public health and provider communities as well as media reporting on LGBTQ issues. Health agencies can consult the CDC about local outbreaks, testing, immunization, and treatment. To get feedback and communicate information to reliable sources, the Biden administration has also spoken with advocates.

To educate gay, bisexual, and other men who have sex with males about monkeypox, the CDC is now offering messaging support to be shared with dating apps.

While noting that the current outbreak has primarily affected men who have sex with men, the CDC and other public health authorities have emphasized that anybody can contract monkeypox in their public communications. The organization has taken care to avoid alienating people who are at higher risk, particularly gay and bisexual men. The CDC advises partners involved in monkeypox messaging to "highlight that anyone can get monkeypox and promote it as a public health concern for all" as one piece of advice.

Focusing on cases involving gay and bisexual men could unintentionally stigmatize this group and give people who are not homosexual and bisexual men a false sense of security. Some members of the LGBTQ+ community have raised worry that efforts to prevent stigmatizing this group may have resulted in the true risk being minimized, leaving the community with insufficient knowledge of monkeypox.

The extent to which state and local health agencies are contacting local providers and severely afflicted populations in addition to the federal government vary, and certain national initiatives, like Greater than AIDS (run by KFF), have created focused messaging for individuals at risk.

What important factors could influence future U.S. outbreak responses?

Numerous factors, including access to testing, vaccination, and treatment, funding and cost issues, community education and messaging, variation in responses across states/jurisdictions, and equity issues, could have an impact on the success of the federal approach to containing and address the current monkeypox outbreak in the United States as reported cases rise.

<u>Access to testing</u>

Early on, some criticized the federal government for failing to set up widespread testing and engage with partners like national pharmacies even though testing is now expanding. The ability to follow the outbreak through testing and provide those who test positive with risk-reduction options including acquiring PEP and stopping further transmission. Additionally, it is a first step toward obtaining treatment, if necessary and practical. Testing can be successfully scaled up if patients and providers are informed about it and barriers like stigma and expense are controlled. While there is now commercial laboratory capacity, it's crucial to keep in mind that not all providers may be able or willing to do sample collection, which could restrict access for individuals. In general, it is unknown if the present testing expansion can keep up with demand within the spreading disease.

Vaccination availability

Additionally, the availability of vaccines has been restricted thus far, and it is unclear how this situation will change over the upcoming months.

Some countries will have quicker access to vaccination than others since distribution is prioritized based on the variables mentioned above. While the federal government's algorithm for distribution is crucial to this, jurisdictional considerations regarding the timing and volume of dose requests to the CDC may also be important. If some jurisdictions take longer than others to request vaccines, this could result in delayed or limited availability of vaccines.

The expediency and consistency of vaccine access across jurisdictions are also impacted by federal and jurisdictional vaccine prioritization and allocation strategies. The current focus on PEP/PEP++ is partly due to the relatively restricted supply of the preferred vaccination and the perception that it is more necessary to address the requirements of individuals who have likely already been exposed. This strategy, however, restricts access for high-risk persons without a known exposure, which may represent a lost chance for disease prevention and assisting in the reduction of new infections. Many jurisdictions have not yet provided a limited supply of PrEP to people who are at higher risk, but some have, including New York City and Washington, D.C.

In many jurisdictions, the demand for vaccinations currently appears to be much higher than the supply. For instance, the D.C. Department of Health in Washington, D.C. opened vaccination appointments at a specific time with a set number of spots (300 in the first instance), and those spots were quickly filled. New York City experienced similar issues, such as the traffic that crashed the city website. Federal and municipal authorities may have a bigger role to play in promoting vaccination once it is more widely used.

Funding Resources and Cost Coverage

Uncertainty exists around how much money may be available for monkeypox under current grants and how much additional money may be required.

The amount of money being used for this purpose should be transparently tracked and reported, as this information can help determine whether more money is required.

In the early stages of the outbreak, the federal government is also paying for some of the costs associated with testing, treatment, and immunization, but it's likely that over time, this arrangement could change. Testing conducted at the CDC or in public health laboratories is currently free of charge for individuals.

Individuals might, however, be responsible for paying test expenses if they use commercial sector labs; the exact cost would depend on insurance coverage. Testing accessibility may be more constrained for those without insurance or with significant cost-sharing requirements for their plan. Currently, immunizations are given out free of charge and are taken from the strategic national stockpile. Similar to that, TPOXX's costs are currently also covered. Individuals could have to pay for doctor visits, hospital stays, and other lab tests that are required for treatment or diagnosis.

Differentiation in Local Reactions

Due to variances in how they are responding to the ongoing monkeypox outbreak (in some cases, for reasons without their control), states and jurisdictions will likely see varying degrees of success in their ability to suppress isolated outbreaks.

The accessibility and distribution of vaccines, distribution strategies (such as PEP or PrEP and to which priority groups), access to local public health testing, particularly for those without insurance, the strength of local response networks, and the availability of funding are among the differences. Depending on a jurisdiction's success in dealing with the outbreak and its capacity to properly communicate with severely affected populations

<u>Equity Challenges</u>

The Biden administration has made health equity a top priority, so efforts to reduce inequalities in access to health information, immunization, and treatment will help stop the outbreak equally among all groups and reach people from all socioeconomic backgrounds (e.g., race, ethnicity, income, etc.).

Health disparities have persisted, as they did with COVID-19 and HIV, and there is a chance that they will do so again in this situation. This happens with immunizations in at least some contexts, according to anecdotal data. Monitoring vaccination and treatment data by race/ethnicity and other demographic variables may help to identify any growing disparities early on since monkeypox vaccination and treatment are now underway, but this data has not yet been made publically available. Targeted outreach, including to people of color and transgender individuals, customized messaging, assuring widespread access to testing, treatment, and vaccination, and relying on reliable messengers are some possible early attempts to address potential inequities.

<u>Kids and the monkeypox</u>

The majority of instances of monkeypox are in adults, but two cases in children in the United States may have made many parents anxious about the hazards for kids.

An infant who is not a US citizen but was tested while visiting Washington, DC, and a toddler from California have been linked to the two new cases of monkeypox in children. Secondary to household transmission or when someone else in the home mistakenly transmits it to a child are these unrelated and isolated patients.

The disease has primarily affected adults so far and spreads through close contact.

It is possible to contract monkeypox by personal contacts, such as a parent hugging or kissing a child, even though intimate contact has been the most common route to contract this illness in this outbreak. The most important factor in determining illness risk is close touch.

Close touch is the primary method of disease transmission.

What may be discovered from uncommon pediatric cases;

Children under the age of eight may be at an elevated risk for serious consequences from monkeypox, according to the Centers for Disease Control and Prevention Trusted Source.

This is probably brought on by a weaker immune system.

It is believed that children and adults both have the same monkeypox symptoms.

There are few specifics about these two kids or how the virus got into them, but it's possible that it was communicated by close touches, such as a parent or guardian embracing or kissing, as well as direct contact with lesions.

Respiratory transmission is also possible, albeit less frequently.

There is currently no protocol for the vaccination of children, although it is theoretically possible for the shot to be effective and accessible. Adults who have been exposed to or are in high-risk circumstances are the only ones who

are eligible for the vaccination.

pregnancy and the monkeypox

The CDC states that there may be an increased risk of serious illness if you contract the infection if you are pregnant or nursing. There is little data on the effects of monkeypox during pregnancy, but according to the WHO, a mother could transmit the virus to her unborn child through the placenta before delivery.

The organ that joins the uterus and the infant is called the placenta (the womb).

This may raise the likelihood of issues like Miscarriages and stillbirths.

There is no information on whether monkeypox can raise the risk of birth abnormalities. But one of the primary signs of monkeypox is fever.

Additionally, a high fever may raise your risk of developing several birth abnormalities if you contract the infection during your first trimester.

Through intimate touch, you could even infect your newborn during or right after delivery. There is no proof, nevertheless, that nursing can transmit the virus.

Inform your doctor right away if you have an infection that has been confirmed. They'll have to keep a careful eye on you and your baby up to delivery. Your doctor may check the baby's heart every two to three days if you are above 26 weeks pregnant or if you are feeling ill.

Until your doctor can check that the baby is growing normally and the placenta is functioning normally, you might also need routine ultrasounds.

If you have monkeypox or suspect you do, your doctor may advise a C-section to lower the chance of infecting the unborn child. Your newborn may be quarantined after birth until there is no longer a risk of infection for their protection.

Regarding prevention, pregnant women have not received special approval for the JYNNEOS monkeypox vaccination. However, a study of 300 pregnant women who received the shot revealed no adverse reactions or miscarriages connected to the immunization. If you have been exposed to the monkeypox virus and are pregnant, trying to get pregnant, or nursing, discuss your options with your doctor.

Can Condoms Aid in Infection Prevention?

Using condoms by themselves is probably not going to stop you from contracting or spreading monkeypox during sex if you or your partner have a monkeypox rash on your genitals or anus.

If you suspect or know you or your partner has the virus, it is much safer to avoid having intercourse. Instead, you could masturbate concurrently while engaging in cybersex via the phone or computer, as long as you kept a minimum of 6 feet between you and your partner.

The CDC advises that if you choose to take the chance of engaging in physical sex, you:

1. Take into account having sex while wearing clothing or while wearing clothing that covers body regions with a rash.
2. Utilize condoms.

3. No kissing.

4. Wash any sex toys or fetish equipment, as
   well as your hands, linens, towels, and
   clothing.

Summary

Despite early criticism, the U.S. response to the monkeypox outbreak has improved over time. However, challenges still exist as the outbreak continues to spread significantly. Particularly, the availability and accessibility of testing, vaccination, and treatment remain constrained and inconsistent nationwide and among various demographic groups. The federal government's capacity to address these issues over the coming months will be a significant factor in determining whether the United States can put an end to the outbreak or risk having monkeypox establish itself as a persistent endemic disease here.

The U.S. has not yet declared this monkeypox outbreak a domestic public health emergency, despite the WHO designating it as a PHEIC. However, the administration is reportedly considering this option. Although it's unclear whether the government will choose to use this lever in the future, doing so would open up several options and give financing access, if necessary.